DIABETES-FRIENDLY RECIPES FOR KIDS TO IMPROVE BLOOD SUGAR CONTROL

Fun & Flavorful Meals for Healthy Blood Sugar

T. John

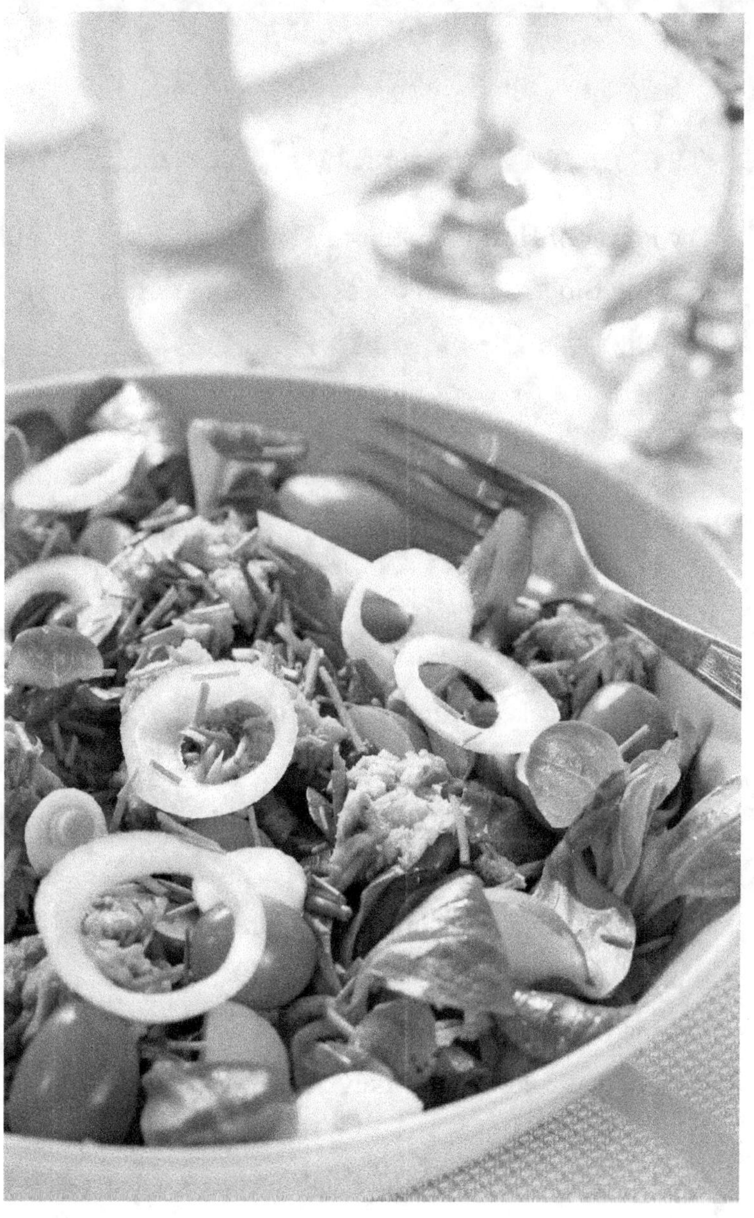

TABLE OF CONTENTS

Chapter 5: Snacks and Appetizers 90

Chapter 6: Desserts 108

INTRODUCTION

I magine this: your energetic child, always on the go, suddenly seems sluggish. Frequent thirst, unusual bathroom habits, and unexplained weight loss might raise concerns. These could be signs of diabetes, a condition that affects how the body uses blood sugar (glucose) for energy.

There are two main types of diabetes that can affect children:

- **Type 1 Diabetes:** In this type, the body doesn't produce enough insulin, a hormone needed to move glucose from the bloodstream into cells.
- **Type 2 Diabetes:** Here, the body either doesn't use insulin effectively or doesn't produce enough.

While the cause of Type 1 diabetes remains unknown, Type 2 is often linked to family history and weight.

The Power of Healthy Eating

Just like any high-octane engine, a growing child's body needs the right fuel. For kids with diabetes, healthy eating becomes even more crucial. Here's why:

- **Balanced Blood Sugar:** Certain foods, like carbohydrates, raise blood sugar levels. A balanced diet with fruits, vegetables, whole grains, and lean protein helps keep blood sugar steady, reducing the highs and lows.
- **Overall Health:** A nutritious diet provides essential vitamins and minerals for development, growth, and a strong immune system to fight off infections.

Making Mealtime a Family Affair:

Involving your child in meal planning and preparation can turn healthy eating into an adventure:

- **Explore the Rainbow:** Fill their plates with a colorful variety of fruits and vegetables. Each color offers a unique set of nutrients!

- **Get Grainy:** Swap refined grains for whole-wheat bread, brown rice, and quinoa. These keep you fuller for longer and provide sustained energy.

- **Supercharge Snacks**: Ditch sugary treats for power-packed alternatives like nuts, yogurt with berries, or carrot sticks with hummus.

- **Be a Role Model:** Healthy eating habits start at home! Make healthy choices yourself and enjoy meals together as a family.

Keeping Blood Sugar in Check

While food plays a starring role, managing blood sugar levels goes hand-in-hand with physical activity:

- **Get Moving:** Encourage your child to find activities they enjoy - bike riding, playing tag, or dancing. Aim for at least 30 minutes of moderate-intensity exercise most days of the week.

- **Plan for Play:** Schedule physical activity around meals and snacks to help regulate blood sugar levels.

- **Team Up for Fun:** Make exercise a family activity! Go for walks, play frisbee in the park, or have a dance party in the living room.

Remember, managing diabetes is a team effort. Your doctor, a registered dietitian, and a diabetes educator can provide guidance and support to create a personalized plan for your child. With a little planning and a lot of love, you can help your child thrive despite diabetes.

Chapter 1: 30 Day Meal Plan

Week 1:

Day 1:

- Breakfast: Oatmeal Pancakes with Fresh Berries
- Lunch: Turkey and Veggie Wrap
- Dinner: Baked Salmon with Asparagus
- Snack: Greek Yogurt Dip with Fresh Veggies
- Dessert: Banana Ice Cream with Dark Chocolate Chips

Day 2:

- Breakfast: Veggie Omelette Muffins
- Lunch: Grilled Chicken Caesar Salad
- Dinner: Turkey Chili with Beans
- Snack: Apple Slices with Almond Butter
- Dessert: Baked Apple Chips

Day 3:

- Breakfast: Whole Wheat French Toast Sticks
- Lunch: Whole Grain Pita Pizza

- Dinner: Cauliflower Crust Veggie Pizza
- Snack: Trail Mix with Nuts and Dried Fruit
- Dessert: Berry Yogurt Popsicles

Day 4:

- Breakfast: Greek Yogurt Parfait with Granola
- Lunch: Quinoa Salad with Roasted Vegetables
- Dinner: Lemon Garlic Chicken with Roasted Vegetables
- Snack: Cottage Cheese with Pineapple Chunks
- Dessert: Chocolate Avocado Mousse

Day 5:

- Breakfast: Spinach and Feta Breakfast Quesadillas
- Lunch: Turkey and Cheese Roll-Ups
- Dinner: Beef and Broccoli Stir-Fry
- Snack: Edamame with Sea Salt
- Dessert: Frozen Grapes

Day 6:

- Breakfast: Banana Walnut Breakfast Cookies
- Lunch: Lentil and Vegetable Soup

- Dinner: Quinoa Stuffed Bell Peppers
- Snack: Guacamole and Baked Tortilla Chips
- Dessert: Mini Fruit Tartlets

Day 7:

- Breakfast: Quinoa Breakfast Bowl with Fruit
- Lunch: Chicken and Vegetable Stir-Fry
- Dinner: Spaghetti Squash with Turkey Bolognese
- Snack: Cucumber and Tomato Salad
- Dessert: Pumpkin Spice Energy Balls

Week 2:

Day 8:

- Breakfast: Breakfast Burrito with Turkey Sausage
- Lunch: Tuna Salad Lettuce Wraps
- Dinner: Grilled Shrimp Skewers with Quinoa
- Snack: Ants on a Log (Celery with Peanut Butter and Raisins)
- Dessert: Strawberry Banana Smoothie Bowl

Day 9:

- Breakfast: Berry Blast Smoothie Bowl

- Lunch: Veggie Hummus Wrap
- Dinner: Veggie Stir-Fry with Tofu
- Snack: Roasted Chickpeas with Seasonings
- Dessert: Yogurt-Dipped Strawberries

Day 10:

- Breakfast: Apple Cinnamon Overnight Oats
- Lunch: Caprese Salad Skewers
- Dinner: Chicken and Vegetable Kebabs
- Snack: Avocado Deviled Eggs
- Dessert: Peach Frozen Yogurt

Day 11:

- Breakfast: Almond Butter Banana Toast
- Lunch: Egg Salad Stuffed Bell Peppers
- Dinner: Black Bean and Corn Quesadillas
- Snack: Whole Grain Pita Chips with Salsa
- Dessert: Blueberry Chia Seed Popsicles

Day 12:

- Breakfast: Veggie Breakfast Casserole
- Lunch: Turkey and Avocado Sandwich

- Dinner: Turkey Meatballs with Zucchini Noodles
- Snack: Turkey and Cheese Kabobs
- Dessert: Watermelon Pizza with Yogurt and Fruit Toppings

Day 13:

- Breakfast: Blueberry Chia Seed Pudding
- Lunch: Baked Sweet Potato Fries
- Dinner: Hawaiian Chicken Kabobs
- Snack: Almond Butter Energy Bites
- Dessert: Mango Sorbet

Day 14:

- Breakfast: Sweet Potato Hash Browns
- Lunch: Greek Couscous Salad
- Dinner: Lentil and Sweet Potato Curry
- Snack: Hummus with Carrot and Celery Sticks
- Dessert: Kiwi and Berry Parfait

Week 3:

Day 15:

- Breakfast: Avocado Toast with Poached Egg

- Lunch: Veggie and Bean Burrito Bowl
- Dinner: Baked Cod with Tomato and Basil
- Snack: Cheese and Whole Grain Crackers
- Dessert: Coconut Almond Date Bites

Day 16:

- Breakfast: Oatmeal Pancakes with Fresh Berries
- Lunch: Turkey and Veggie Wrap
- Dinner: Baked Salmon with Asparagus
- Snack: Apple Slices with Almond Butter
- Dessert: Banana Ice Cream with Dark Chocolate Chips

Day 17:

- Breakfast: Veggie Omelette Muffins
- Lunch: Grilled Chicken Caesar Salad
- Dinner: Turkey Chili with Beans
- Snack: Greek Yogurt Dip with Fresh Veggies
- Dessert: Baked Apple Chips

Day 18:

- Breakfast: Whole Wheat French Toast Sticks

- Lunch: Whole Grain Pita Pizza
- Dinner: Cauliflower Crust Veggie Pizza
- Snack: Trail Mix with Nuts and Dried Fruit
- Dessert: Berry Yogurt Popsicles

Day 19:

- Breakfast: Greek Yogurt Parfait with Granola
- Lunch: Quinoa Salad with Roasted Vegetables
- Dinner: Lemon Garlic Chicken with Roasted Vegetables
- Snack: Cottage Cheese with Pineapple Chunks
- Dessert: Chocolate Avocado Mousse

Day 20:

- Breakfast: Spinach and Feta Breakfast Quesadillas
- Lunch: Turkey and Cheese Roll-Ups
- Dinner: Beef and Broccoli Stir-Fry
- Snack: Edamame with Sea Salt
- Dessert: Frozen Grapes

Day 21:

- Breakfast: Banana Walnut Breakfast Cookies

- Lunch: Lentil and Vegetable Soup

- Dinner: Quinoa Stuffed Bell Peppers

- Snack: Guacamole and Baked Tortilla Chips

- Dessert: Mini Fruit Tartlets

Week 4:

Day 22:

- Breakfast: Quinoa Breakfast Bowl with Fruit

- Lunch: Chicken and Vegetable Stir-Fry

- Dinner: Spaghetti Squash with Turkey Bolognese

- Snack: Cucumber and Tomato Salad

- Dessert: Pumpkin Spice Energy Balls

Day 23:

- Breakfast: Breakfast Burrito with Turkey Sausage

- Lunch: Tuna Salad Lettuce Wraps

- Dinner: Grilled Shrimp Skewers with Quinoa

- Snack: Ants on a Log (Celery with Peanut Butter and Raisins)

- Dessert: Strawberry Banana Smoothie Bowl

Day 24:

- Breakfast: Berry Blast Smoothie Bowl
- Lunch: Veggie Hummus Wrap
- Dinner: Veggie Stir-Fry with Tofu
- Snack: Roasted Chickpeas with Seasonings
- Dessert: Yogurt-Dipped Strawberries

Day 25:

- Breakfast: Apple Cinnamon Overnight Oats
- Lunch: Caprese Salad Skewers
- Dinner: Chicken and Vegetable Kebabs
- Snack: Avocado Deviled Eggs
- Dessert: Peach Frozen Yogurt

Day 26:

- Breakfast: Almond Butter Banana Toast
- Lunch: Egg Salad Stuffed Bell Peppers
- Dinner: Black Bean and Corn Quesadillas
- Snack: Whole Grain Pita Chips with Salsa
- Dessert: Blueberry Chia Seed Popsicles

Day 27:

- Breakfast: Veggie Breakfast Casserole
- Lunch: Turkey and Avocado Sandwich
- Dinner: Turkey Meatballs with Zucchini Noodles
- Snack: Turkey and Cheese Kabobs
- Dessert: Watermelon Pizza with Yogurt and Fruit Toppings

Day 28:

- Breakfast: Blueberry Chia Seed Pudding
- Lunch: Baked Sweet Potato Fries
- Dinner: Hawaiian Chicken Kabobs
- Snack: Almond Butter Energy Bites
- Dessert: Mango Sorbet

Day 29:

- Breakfast: Sweet Potato Hash Browns
- Lunch: Greek Couscous Salad
- Dinner: Lentil and Sweet Potato Curry
- Snack: Hummus with Carrot and Celery Sticks
- Dessert: Kiwi and Berry Parfait

Day 30:

- Breakfast: Avocado Toast with Poached Egg
- Lunch: Veggie and Bean Burrito Bowl
- Dinner: Baked Cod with Tomato and Basil
- Snack: Cheese and Whole Grain Crackers
- Dessert: Coconut Almond Date Bites

Chapter 2: Breakfast Recipes

These recipes are designed to help regulate blood sugar levels while still providing the essential nutrients and energy needed to fuel busy mornings. From hearty pancakes to satisfying smoothie bowls, there's something here to please every palate.

Oatmeal Pancakes with Fresh Berries

Ingredients:

- 1 cup rolled oats
- 1 ripe banana, mashed
- 2 eggs
- 1/2 teaspoon vanilla extract
- 1/2 teaspoon cinnamon
- 1/4 cup fresh berries (strawberries, blueberries, raspberries)

Instructions:

1. In a blender, combine rolled oats, mashed banana, eggs, vanilla extract, and cinnamon. Blend until smooth.
2. Heat a non-stick skillet over medium heat and lightly grease with cooking spray.
3. Pour pancake batter onto the skillet to form small pancakes.
4. Cook for 2-3 minutes on each side, until golden brown.
5. Serve pancakes topped with fresh berries.

Nutrition Information (per serving):

- Calories: 250
- Protein: 10g
- Carbohydrates: 40g
- Fat: 6g
- Fiber: 6g
- Sugar: 10g
- Portion Size: 2 pancakes

Veggie Omelette Muffins

Ingredients:

- 6 eggs
- 1/4 cup diced bell peppers
- 1/4 cup diced onions
- 1/4 cup diced tomatoes
- Salt and pepper, to taste

Instructions:

1. Preheat oven to 350°F (175°C) and grease a muffin tin with cooking spray.
2. In a bowl, whisk together eggs, bell peppers, onions, tomatoes, salt, and pepper.
3. Pour egg mixture into muffin tin, filling each cup about 3/4 full.
4. Bake for 15-20 minutes, until eggs are set and lightly golden.
5. Allow muffins to cool slightly before serving.

Nutrition Information (per serving - 2 muffins):

- Calories: 180
- Protein: 14g

- Carbohydrates: 4g
- Fat: 12g
- Fiber: 1g
- Sugar: 2g
- Portion Size: 2 muffins

Whole Wheat French Toast Sticks

Ingredients:

- 4 slices whole wheat bread
- 2 eggs
- 1/4 cup milk (or almond milk)
- 1/2 teaspoon cinnamon
- 1/4 teaspoon vanilla extract

Instructions:

1. Cut each slice of bread into strips to make sticks.
2. In a shallow bowl, whisk together eggs, milk, cinnamon, and vanilla extract.
3. Dip bread sticks into egg mixture, coating evenly.
4. Heat a non-stick skillet over medium heat and lightly grease with cooking spray.

5. Cook bread sticks for 2-3 minutes on each side, until golden brown.

6. Serve warm with a side of sugar-free syrup or fresh fruit.

Nutrition Information (per serving):

- Calories: 180

- Protein: 9g

- Carbohydrates: 20g

- Fat: 7g

- Fiber: 4g

- Sugar: 3g

- Portion Size: 4 French toast sticks

Greek Yogurt Parfait with Granola

Ingredients:

- 1/2 cup Greek yogurt

- 1/4 cup granola (sugar-free or low-sugar)

- 1/4 cup mixed berries (strawberries, blueberries, raspberries)

Instructions:

1. In a glass or bowl, layer Greek yogurt, granola, and mixed berries.
2. Repeat layers until ingredients are used up.
3. Serve immediately or refrigerate for later.

Nutrition Information (per serving):

- Calories: 200
- Protein: 12g
- Carbohydrates: 25g
- Fat: 6g
- Fiber: 4g
- Sugar: 10g
- Portion Size: 1 parfait

Spinach and Feta Breakfast Quesadillas

Ingredients:

- 2 whole wheat tortillas
- 1/2 cup fresh spinach leaves
- 1/4 cup crumbled feta cheese

- 2 eggs, scrambled

Instructions:

1. Heat a non-stick skillet over medium heat and lightly grease with cooking spray.
2. Place one tortilla in the skillet and top with spinach, feta cheese, and scrambled eggs.
3. Place the second tortilla on top like a sandwich.
4. Cook for 2-3 minutes on each side, until tortillas are golden brown and cheese is melted.
5. Cut quesadilla into wedges and serve hot.

Nutrition Information (per serving):

- Calories: 280
- Protein: 16g
- Carbohydrates: 20g
- Fat: 14g
- Fiber: 4g
- Sugar: 2g
- Portion Size: 1 quesadilla

Banana Walnut Breakfast Cookies

Ingredients:

- 2 ripe bananas, mashed
- 1 cup old-fashioned oats
- 1/4 cup chopped walnuts
- 1/4 cup raisins
- 1 teaspoon cinnamon

Instructions:

1. Preheat oven to 350°F (175°C) and line a baking sheet with parchment paper.
2. In a bowl, combine mashed bananas, oats, walnuts, raisins, and cinnamon.
3. Mix until well combined.
4. Drop spoonfuls of the mixture onto the prepared baking sheet and flatten slightly with the back of a spoon.
5. Bake for 15-20 minutes, until cookies are golden brown.
6. Allow cookies to cool before serving.

Nutrition Information (per serving - 2 cookies):

- Calories: 180

- Protein: 4g

- Carbohydrates: 30g

- Fat: 6g

- Fiber: 4g

- Sugar: 12g

- Portion Size: 2 cookies

Quinoa Breakfast Bowl with Fruit

Ingredients:

- 1/2 cup cooked quinoa

- 1/4 cup sliced strawberries

- 1/4 cup blueberries

- 1 tablespoon honey (optional)

- 1 tablespoon chopped nuts (almonds, walnuts, or pecans)

Instructions:

1. In a bowl, layer cooked quinoa, sliced strawberries, and blueberries.

2. Drizzle with honey, if desired, and sprinkle with chopped nuts.

3. Serve immediately.

Nutrition Information (per serving):

- Calories: 220

- Protein: 6g

- Carbohydrates: 40g

- Fat: 5g

- Fiber: 6g

- Sugar: 15g

- Portion Size: 1 bowl

Breakfast Burrito with Turkey Sausage

Ingredients:

- 2 whole wheat tortillas

- 2 turkey sausage links, cooked and sliced

- 2 eggs, scrambled

- 1/4 cup shredded cheddar cheese

- Salsa or hot sauce (optional)

Instructions:

1. Heat a non-stick skillet over medium heat and lightly grease with cooking spray.
2. Place tortillas in the skillet and top with cooked turkey sausage, scrambled eggs, and shredded cheddar cheese.
3. Roll up tortillas into burritos and cook for 2-3 minutes on each side, until heated through and cheese is melted.
4. Serve hot with salsa or hot sauce, if desired.

Nutrition Information (per serving):

- Calories: 320
- Protein: 20g
- Carbohydrates: 25g
- Fat: 16g
- Fiber: 4g
- Sugar: 2g
- Portion Size: 1 burrito

Berry Blast Smoothie Bowl

Ingredients:

- 1 cup frozen mixed berries (strawberries, blueberries, raspberries)
- 1/2 banana
- 1/2 cup Greek yogurt
- 1/4 cup almond milk (or any milk of choice)
- 1 tablespoon honey (optional)
- Toppings: sliced banana, granola, chia seeds, shredded coconut

Instructions:

1. In a blender, combine frozen mixed berries, banana, Greek yogurt, almond milk, and honey.
2. Blend until smooth and creamy, adding more milk if needed to reach desired consistency.
3. Pour smoothie into a bowl and top with sliced banana, granola, chia seeds, and shredded coconut.
4. Serve immediately.

Nutrition Information (per serving):

- Calories: 250

- Protein: 10g

- Carbohydrates: 40g

- Fat: 6g

- Fiber: 8g

- Sugar: 25g

- Portion Size: 1 bowl

Apple Cinnamon Overnight Oats

Ingredients:

- 1/2 cup rolled oats

- 1/2 cup unsweetened applesauce

- 1/2 cup almond milk (or any milk of choice)

- 1 tablespoon maple syrup (or honey)

- 1/2 teaspoon cinnamon

- 1/4 cup diced apples

- 1 tablespoon chopped nuts (walnuts or almonds)

Instructions:

1. In a jar or container, combine rolled oats, applesauce, almond milk, maple syrup, and cinnamon.

2. Stir in diced apples and chopped nuts.

3. Cover and refrigerate overnight.

4. In the morning, stir well and add a splash of milk if needed to reach desired consistency.

5. Serve cold or warm, as desired.

Nutrition Information (per serving):

- Calories: 280
- Protein: 6g
- Carbohydrates: 45g
- Fat: 8g
- Fiber: 7g
- Sugar: 20g
- Portion Size: 1 serving

Almond Butter Banana Toast

Ingredients:

- 2 slices whole wheat bread, toasted
- 2 tablespoons almond butter
- 1 banana, sliced
- 1 tablespoon honey (optional)
- Pinch of cinnamon

Instructions:

1. Spread almond butter evenly on toasted whole wheat bread slices.
2. Top with sliced banana.
3. Drizzle with honey, if desired, and sprinkle with a pinch of cinnamon.
4. Serve immediately.

Nutrition Information (per serving):

- Calories: 320
- Protein: 8g
- Carbohydrates: 45g
- Fat: 14g
- Fiber: 8g
- Sugar: 15g
- Portion Size: 2 slices of toast

Veggie Breakfast Casserole

Ingredients:

- 6 eggs
- 1/2 cup milk (or almond milk)

- 1 cup chopped mixed vegetables (bell peppers, onions, spinach)
- 1/2 cup shredded cheddar cheese
- Salt and pepper, to taste

Instructions:

1. Preheat oven to 350°F (175°C) and grease a baking dish with cooking spray.
2. In a bowl, whisk together eggs, milk, salt, and pepper.
3. Stir in chopped mixed vegetables and shredded cheddar cheese.
4. Pour mixture into the prepared baking dish.
5. Bake for 25-30 minutes, until eggs are set and edges are golden brown.
6. Allow casserole to cool slightly before slicing and serving.

Nutrition Information (per serving):

- Calories: 200
- Protein: 15g
- Carbohydrates: 5g

- Fat: 12g

- Fiber: 1g

- Sugar: 2g

- Portion Size: 1 serving

Blueberry Chia Seed Pudding

Ingredients:

- 1/4 cup chia seeds

- 1 cup almond milk (or any milk of choice)

- 1/2 cup fresh blueberries

- 1 tablespoon honey (optional)

- 1/2 teaspoon vanilla extract

Instructions:

1. In a jar or bowl, mix together chia seeds, almond milk, honey, and vanilla extract.

2. Stir in fresh blueberries.

3. Cover and refrigerate for at least 2 hours or overnight, until pudding has thickened.

4. Stir well before serving.

5. Serve chilled, topped with additional blueberries if desired.

Nutrition Information (per serving):

- Calories: 180
- Protein: 5g
- Carbohydrates: 20g
- Fat: 9g
- Fiber: 9g
- Sugar: 8g
- Portion Size: 1 serving

Sweet Potato Hash Browns

Ingredients:

- 2 medium sweet potatoes, grated
- 1/4 cup onion, finely chopped
- 1 tablespoon olive oil
- Salt and pepper, to taste

Instructions:

1. Heat olive oil in a skillet over medium heat.
2. Add grated sweet potatoes and chopped onion to the skillet.
3. Season with salt and pepper, to taste.

4. Cook for 10-12 minutes, stirring occasionally, until sweet potatoes are tender and golden brown.

5. Serve hot as a side dish or as a base for other breakfast items.

Nutrition Information (per serving):

- Calories: 150

- Protein: 2g

- Carbohydrates: 20g

- Fat: 7g

- Fiber: 3g

- Sugar: 5g

- Portion Size: 1 serving

Avocado Toast with Poached Egg

Ingredients:

- 2 slices whole grain bread, toasted

- 1 ripe avocado, mashed

- 2 eggs, poached

- Salt and pepper, to taste

- Red pepper flakes (optional)

Instructions:

1. Spread mashed avocado evenly on toasted whole grain bread slices.

2. Top each slice with a poached egg.

3. Season with salt, pepper, and red pepper flakes, if desired.

4. Serve immediately.

Nutrition Information (per serving):

- Calories: 300

- Protein: 14g

- Carbohydrates: 20g

- Fat: 20g

- Fiber: 7g

- Sugar: 2g

- Portion Size: 2 slices of toast

Chapter 3: Lunch Recipes

In this chapter, we present a delightful array of lunch recipes that are not only delicious but also packed with wholesome goodness. From wraps to salads to hearty soups, there's something here to satisfy every palate. Each recipe is crafted with care to provide balanced nutrition, making them perfect for a midday meal that will keep you feeling satisfied and fueled for the day ahead.

Turkey and Veggie Wrap

Ingredients:

- Whole wheat tortilla
- Sliced turkey breast
- Sliced cucumbers
- Shredded carrots
- Spinach leaves
- Hummus

Instructions:

1. Lay the tortilla flat and spread a layer of hummus over it.

2. Arrange the turkey slices, cucumbers, shredded carrots, and spinach leaves on top of the hummus.

3. Roll the tortilla tightly, enclosing the fillings.

4. Slice the wrap in half diagonally.

5. Serve and enjoy!

Nutrition Information:

- Calories: 280

- Protein: 18g

- Carbohydrates: 35g

- Fat: 8g

- Fiber: 6g

- Sugar: 4g

- Portion Size: 1 wrap

Grilled Chicken Caesar Salad

Ingredients:

- Grilled chicken breast, sliced

- Romaine lettuce, chopped

- Cherry tomatoes, halved
- Grated Parmesan cheese
- Whole wheat croutons
- Caesar dressing

Instructions:

1. In a large bowl, combine the chopped romaine lettuce, cherry tomatoes, and grilled chicken slices.
2. Add the grated Parmesan cheese and whole wheat croutons.
3. Drizzle Caesar dressing over the salad.
4. Toss until well combined.
5. Serve immediately.

Nutrition Information:

- Calories: 320
- Protein: 25g
- Carbohydrates: 15g
- Fat: 18g
- Fiber: 5g
- Sugar: 3g
- Portion Size: 1 serving

Whole Grain Pita Pizza

Ingredients:

- Whole grain pita bread
- Tomato sauce
- Shredded mozzarella cheese
- Sliced bell peppers
- Sliced mushrooms
- Sliced black olives

Instructions:

1. Preheat the oven to 375°F (190°C).
2. Place the whole grain pita bread on a baking sheet.
3. Spread tomato sauce over the pita bread.
4. Sprinkle shredded mozzarella cheese over the sauce.
5. Arrange sliced bell peppers, mushrooms, and black olives on top.
6. Bake in the preheated oven for 10-12 minutes, or until the cheese is melted and bubbly.
7. Remove from the oven and slice.
8. Serve hot.

Nutrition Information:

- Calories: 240
- Protein: 12g
- Carbohydrates: 30g
- Fat: 9g
- Fiber: 5g
- Sugar: 4g
- Portion Size: 1 pizza

Quinoa Salad with Roasted Vegetables

Ingredients:

- Quinoa
- Assorted vegetables (such as bell peppers, zucchini, and cherry tomatoes)
- Olive oil
- Balsamic vinegar
- Fresh herbs (such as parsley or basil)
- Salt and pepper to taste

Instructions:

1. Cook quinoa according to package instructions and let it cool.
2. Preheat the oven to 400°F (200°C).
3. Chop the vegetables into bite-sized pieces and place them on a baking sheet.
4. Drizzle with olive oil and balsamic vinegar, then season with salt and pepper.
5. Roast in the preheated oven for 20-25 minutes or until the vegetables are tender and slightly caramelized.
6. In a large bowl, combine the cooked quinoa with the roasted vegetables.
7. Garnish with fresh herbs.
8. Serve as a nutritious salad.

Nutrition Information:

- Calories: 280
- Protein: 8g
- Carbohydrates: 40g
- Fat: 10g
- Fiber: 6g

- Sugar: 5g
- Portion Size: 1 cup

Turkey and Cheese Roll-Ups

Ingredients:

- Deli turkey slices
- Cheese slices (such as cheddar or Swiss)
- Spinach leaves
- Mustard or mayonnaise (optional)

Instructions:

1. Lay a turkey slice flat and place a cheese slice on top.
2. Add a few spinach leaves on one end of the turkey slice.
3. Roll the turkey slice tightly, enclosing the spinach and cheese.
4. Secure with toothpicks if necessary.
5. Repeat with remaining turkey slices and cheese.
6. Optionally, serve with mustard or mayonnaise for dipping.
7. Enjoy these tasty roll-ups!

Nutrition Information:

- Calories: 200
- Protein: 15g
- Carbohydrates: 2g
- Fat: 15g
- Fiber: 1g
- Sugar: 1g
- Portion Size: 2 roll-ups

Lentil and Vegetable Soup

Ingredients:

- Green lentils
- Assorted vegetables (such as carrots, celery, and onions)
- Vegetable broth
- Garlic, minced
- Bay leaf
- Salt and pepper to taste

Instructions:

1. Rinse the lentils and set them aside.
2. In a large pot, heat some olive oil over medium heat.

3. Add minced garlic and sauté until fragrant.

4. Add chopped vegetables and cook until softened.

5. Pour in the vegetable broth and add the bay leaf.

6. Bring the mixture to a boil, then reduce heat and simmer for 20-25 minutes, or until the lentils are tender.

7. Season with salt and pepper to taste.

8. Serve hot as a comforting and nutritious lunch option.

Nutrition Information:

- Calories: 220
- Protein: 12g
- Carbohydrates: 35g
- Fat: 3g
- Fiber: 10g
- Sugar: 5g
- Portion Size: 1 cup

Chicken and Vegetable Stir-Fry

Ingredients:

- Chicken breast, sliced

- Assorted vegetables (such as bell peppers, broccoli, and snap peas)
- Soy sauce
- Garlic, minced
- Ginger, grated
- Sesame oil
- Cooked brown rice or quinoa

Instructions:

1. Heat sesame oil in a large skillet or wok over medium-high heat.
2. Add minced garlic and grated ginger, and stir-fry for about 30 seconds.
3. Add sliced chicken breast and cook until no longer pink.
4. Add assorted vegetables and continue stir-frying until they are crisp-tender.
5. Drizzle soy sauce over the stir-fry and toss to coat evenly.
6. Serve hot over cooked brown rice or quinoa.

Nutrition Information:

- Calories: 300
- Protein: 25g
- Carbohydrates: 30g
- Fat: 8g
- Fiber: 6g
- Sugar: 4g
- Portion Size: 1 cup stir-fry with 1/2 cup cooked rice/quinoa

Tuna Salad Lettuce Wraps

Ingredients:

- Canned tuna, drained
- Greek yogurt
- Diced celery
- Diced red onion
- Diced bell pepper
- Lemon juice
- Salt and pepper to taste
- Lettuce leaves for wrapping

Instructions:

1. In a bowl, mix together canned tuna, Greek yogurt, diced celery, red onion, and bell pepper.

2. Add lemon juice, salt, and pepper to taste, and mix well.

3. Spoon the tuna salad onto lettuce leaves.

4. Wrap the lettuce leaves around the tuna salad, securing with toothpicks if needed.

5. Serve chilled and enjoy these refreshing lettuce wraps.

Nutrition Information:

- Calories: 150
- Protein: 20g
- Carbohydrates: 5g
- Fat: 6g
- Fiber: 2g
- Sugar: 2g
- Portion Size: 2 lettuce wraps

Veggie Hummus Wrap

Ingredients:

- Whole wheat tortilla
- Hummus
- Sliced cucumber
- Sliced bell pepper
- Shredded carrots
- Spinach leaves

Instructions:

1. Spread hummus evenly over the whole wheat tortilla.
2. Layer sliced cucumber, bell pepper, shredded carrots, and spinach leaves on top of the hummus.
3. Roll the tortilla tightly, enclosing the vegetables.
4. Cut the wrap in half diagonally.
5. Serve and enjoy this nutritious and flavorful veggie wrap.

Nutrition Information:

- Calories: 220
- Protein: 8g
- Carbohydrates: 35g

- Fat: 7g

- Fiber: 8g

- Sugar: 4g

- Portion Size: 1 wrap

Caprese Salad Skewers

Ingredients:

- Cherry tomatoes

- Fresh mozzarella balls

- Fresh basil leaves

- Balsamic glaze

- Skewers

Instructions:

1. Thread a cherry tomato, a mozzarella ball, and a basil leaf onto each skewer.

2. Arrange the skewers on a serving platter.

3. Drizzle with balsamic glaze.

4. Serve as a delightful and refreshing salad option.

Nutrition Information:

- Calories: 120

- Protein: 6g

- Carbohydrates: 4g

- Fat: 8g

- Fiber: 1g

- Sugar: 2g

- Portion Size: 2 skewers

Egg Salad Stuffed Bell Peppers

Ingredients:

- Hard-boiled eggs, chopped

- Greek yogurt

- Dijon mustard

- Chopped celery

- Chopped red onion

- Chopped parsley

- Salt and pepper to taste

- Bell peppers, halved and deseeded

Instructions:

1. In a bowl, mix together chopped hard-boiled eggs, Greek yogurt, Dijon mustard, celery, red onion, parsley, salt, and pepper.

2. Spoon the egg salad mixture into halved bell peppers.

3. Serve chilled or at room temperature as a delicious and protein-packed lunch option.

Nutrition Information:

- Calories: 180
- Protein: 12g
- Carbohydrates: 8g
- Fat: 10g
- Fiber: 2g
- Sugar: 4g
- Portion Size: 1 stuffed bell pepper

Turkey and Avocado Sandwich

Ingredients:

- Whole grain bread slices
- Sliced turkey breast
- Avocado, mashed
- Tomato slices
- Lettuce leaves
- Mustard or mayonnaise (optional)

Instructions:

1. Spread mashed avocado on one slice of whole grain bread.
2. Layer sliced turkey breast, tomato slices, and lettuce leaves on top.
3. Optionally, spread mustard or mayonnaise on the other slice of bread before placing it on top.
4. Cut the sandwich in half diagonally.
5. Serve and enjoy this hearty and nutritious sandwich.

Nutrition Information:

- Calories: 320
- Protein: 20g
- Carbohydrates: 25g
- Fat: 15g
- Fiber: 8g
- Sugar: 4g
- Portion Size: 1 sandwich

Baked Sweet Potato Fries

Ingredients:

- Sweet potatoes, peeled and cut into fries

- Olive oil

- Salt and pepper to taste

- Optional: seasoning of choice (such as paprika or garlic powder)

Instructions:

1. Preheat the oven to 425°F (220°C) and line a baking sheet with parchment paper.

2. Toss sweet potato fries with olive oil, salt, pepper, and any optional seasoning of choice until evenly coated.

3. Spread the fries in a single layer on the prepared baking sheet.

4. Bake for 20-25 minutes, flipping halfway through, or until the fries are crispy and golden brown.

5. Remove from the oven and serve hot as a delicious and nutritious side dish.

Nutrition Information:

- Calories: 150

- Protein: 2g

- Carbohydrates: 25g

- Fat: 5g

- Fiber: 4g

- Sugar: 5g

- Portion Size: 1 cup of fries

Greek Couscous Salad

Ingredients:

- Couscous

- Cherry tomatoes, halved

- Cucumber, diced

- Red onion, finely chopped

- Kalamata olives, pitted and sliced

- Feta cheese, crumbled

- Fresh parsley, chopped

- Lemon juice

- Extra virgin olive oil

- Salt and pepper to taste

Instructions:

1. Cook couscous according to package instructions and let it cool.

2. In a large bowl, combine the cooked couscous, cherry tomatoes, cucumber, red onion, olives, feta cheese, and parsley.

3. Drizzle with lemon juice and extra virgin olive oil.

4. Season with salt and pepper to taste.

5. Toss until well combined.

6. Serve chilled as a refreshing and flavorful salad option.

Nutrition Information:

- Calories: 280
- Protein: 8g
- Carbohydrates: 35g
- Fat: 12g
- Fiber: 5g
- Sugar: 4g
- Portion Size: 1 cup

Veggie and Bean Burrito Bowl

Ingredients:

- Cooked brown rice
- Black beans, drained and rinsed

- Corn kernels
- Diced bell peppers
- Diced tomatoes
- Avocado, sliced
- Fresh cilantro, chopped
- Lime wedges
- Salsa (optional)

Instructions:

1. In individual serving bowls, layer cooked brown rice, black beans, corn kernels, diced bell peppers, and diced tomatoes.
2. Top with sliced avocado and chopped cilantro.
3. Serve with lime wedges and salsa on the side, if desired.
4. Enjoy this hearty and flavorful burrito bowl as a nutritious lunch option.

Nutrition Information:

- Calories: 320
- Protein: 10g
- Carbohydrates: 50g

- Fat: 10g
- Fiber: 12g
- Sugar: 5g
- Portion Size: 1 bowl

Chapter 4: Dinner Recipes

These dinner recipes are not only delicious but also packed with nutritious ingredients to support overall health and well-being. From hearty proteins to fiber-rich vegetables, each recipe is carefully crafted to provide a balanced and satisfying meal that the whole family will love.

Baked Salmon with Asparagus

Ingredients:

- 4 salmon fillets
- 1 bunch of asparagus
- Olive oil
- Lemon juice
- Garlic powder
- Salt and pepper

Instructions:

1. Preheat the oven to 400°F (200°C).
2. Place salmon fillets on a baking sheet lined with parchment paper.

3. Arrange asparagus spears around the salmon.

4. Drizzle olive oil and lemon juice over the salmon and asparagus.

5. Sprinkle with garlic powder, salt, and pepper.

6. Bake for 12-15 minutes until salmon is cooked through and asparagus is tender.

7. Serve hot.

Nutrition Information:

- Calories: 300
- Protein: 25g
- Carbohydrates: 5g
- Fat: 20g
- Fiber: 2g
- Sugar: 2g
- Portion size: 1 fillet of salmon with asparagus

Turkey Chili with Beans

Ingredients:

- 1 lb ground turkey
- 1 can kidney beans, drained and rinsed
- 1 can diced tomatoes

- 1 onion, diced
- 2 cloves garlic, minced
- 1 tablespoon chili powder
- 1 teaspoon cumin
- Salt and pepper to taste

Instructions:

1. In a large pot, cook ground turkey over medium heat until browned.
2. Add diced onions and garlic, cook until softened.
3. Stir in diced tomatoes, kidney beans, chili powder, cumin, salt, and pepper.
4. Simmer for 20-25 minutes, stirring occasionally.
5. Serve hot.

Nutrition Information:

- Calories: 280
- Protein: 22g
- Carbohydrates: 20g
- Fat: 10g
- Fiber: 6g
- Sugar: 4g

- Portion size: 1 cup

Cauliflower Crust Veggie Pizza

Ingredients:

- 1 cauliflower crust (store-bought or homemade)
- 1 cup marinara sauce
- 1 cup shredded mozzarella cheese
- Assorted vegetables (bell peppers, mushrooms, onions, tomatoes)

Instructions:

1. Preheat the oven according to the cauliflower crust package instructions.
2. Spread marinara sauce over the cauliflower crust.
3. Sprinkle shredded mozzarella cheese on top.
4. Arrange assorted vegetables over the cheese.
5. Bake for 10-15 minutes until cheese is melted and bubbly.
6. Slice and serve hot.

Nutrition Information:

- Calories: 200

- Protein: 10g
- Carbohydrates: 15g
- Fat: 10g
- Fiber: 5g
- Sugar: 5g
- Portion size: 1 slice (1/6 of pizza)

Lemon Garlic Chicken with Roasted Vegetables

Ingredients:

- 4 chicken breasts
- 2 cups mixed vegetables (bell peppers, zucchini, carrots)
- 2 tablespoons olive oil
- 2 cloves garlic, minced
- Zest and juice of 1 lemon
- Salt and pepper to taste

Instructions:

1. Preheat the oven to 400°F (200°C).

2. Place chicken breasts and mixed vegetables on a baking sheet.

3. In a small bowl, whisk together olive oil, minced garlic, lemon zest, lemon juice, salt, and pepper.

4. Drizzle the lemon garlic mixture over the chicken and vegetables.

5. Roast in the oven for 20-25 minutes until chicken is cooked through and vegetables are tender.

6. Serve hot.

Nutrition Information:

- Calories: 280
- Protein: 30g
- Carbohydrates: 10g
- Fat: 12g
- Fiber: 4g
- Sugar: 4g
- Portion size: 1 chicken breast with roasted vegetables

Beef and Broccoli Stir-Fry

Ingredients:

- 1 lb beef sirloin, thinly sliced

- 2 cups broccoli florets
- 1 bell pepper, sliced
- 1 onion, sliced
- 2 cloves garlic, minced
- 1/4 cup low-sodium soy sauce
- 2 tablespoons hoisin sauce
- 1 tablespoon cornstarch
- 1 tablespoon sesame oil

Instructions:

1. In a small bowl, whisk together soy sauce, hoisin sauce, and cornstarch.
2. Heat sesame oil in a large skillet over medium-high heat.
3. Add minced garlic and sliced beef to the skillet, cook until beef is browned.
4. Add broccoli florets, bell pepper, and onion to the skillet, stir-fry for 3-4 minutes.
5. Pour the sauce mixture over the beef and vegetables, stir well to combine.
6. Cook for another 2-3 minutes until sauce thickens.
7. Serve hot over cooked rice or quinoa.

Nutrition Information:

- Calories: 320
- Protein: 25g
- Carbohydrates: 15g
- Fat: 18g
- Fiber: 4g
- Sugar: 6g
- Portion size: 1 cup of stir-fry with rice or quinoa

Quinoa Stuffed Bell Peppers

Ingredients:

- 4 bell peppers, halved and seeds removed
- 1 cup quinoa, cooked
- 1 can black beans, drained and rinsed
- 1 cup diced tomatoes
- 1/2 cup corn kernels
- 1/4 cup chopped cilantro
- 1 teaspoon cumin
- Salt and pepper to taste
- Shredded cheese for topping (optional)

Instructions:

1. Preheat the oven to 375°F (190°C).
2. In a large bowl, combine cooked quinoa, black beans, diced tomatoes, corn kernels, chopped cilantro, cumin, salt, and pepper.
3. Stuff the halved bell peppers with the quinoa mixture.
4. Place stuffed bell peppers in a baking dish.
5. Cover the dish with foil and bake for 25-30 minutes.
6. Remove foil, sprinkle shredded cheese on top (if using), and bake for an additional 5 minutes until cheese is melted.
7. Serve hot.

Nutrition Information:

- Calories: 250
- Protein: 12g
- Carbohydrates: 40g
- Fat: 5g
- Fiber: 8g
- Sugar: 6g
- Portion size: 1 stuffed bell pepper half

Spaghetti Squash with Turkey Bolognese

Ingredients:

- 1 spaghetti squash
- 1 lb ground turkey
- 1 can crushed tomatoes
- 1 onion, diced
- 2 cloves garlic, minced
- 1 teaspoon Italian seasoning
- Salt and pepper to taste
- Fresh basil leaves for garnish

Instructions:

1. Preheat the oven to 400°F (200°C).
2. Cut the spaghetti squash in half lengthwise and scoop out the seeds.
3. Place the squash halves cut side down on a baking sheet lined with parchment paper.
4. Bake for 30-40 minutes until squash is tender.
5. Meanwhile, in a large skillet, cook ground turkey over medium heat until browned.

6. Add diced onions and minced garlic, cook until softened.

7. Stir in crushed tomatoes, Italian seasoning, salt, and pepper. Simmer for 10-15 minutes.

8. Use a fork to scrape the spaghetti squash into strands.

9. Serve the turkey bolognese sauce over the spaghetti squash strands.

10. Garnish with fresh basil leaves.

Nutrition Information:

- Calories: 280
- Protein: 25g
- Carbohydrates: 20g
- Fat: 10g
- Fiber: 6g
- Sugar: 8g
- Portion size: 1 cup of spaghetti squash with sauce

Grilled Shrimp Skewers with Quinoa

Ingredients:

- 1 lb shrimp, peeled and deveined
- 2 cups cooked quinoa

- 1 bell pepper, diced
- 1 zucchini, diced
- 1 lemon, sliced
- 2 tablespoons olive oil
- 1 teaspoon paprika
- Salt and pepper to taste
- Wooden skewers, soaked in water

Instructions:

1. Preheat the grill to medium-high heat.
2. Thread shrimp, diced bell pepper, and diced zucchini onto the wooden skewers.
3. Drizzle olive oil over the skewers and sprinkle with paprika, salt, and pepper.
4. Grill the skewers for 2-3 minutes on each side until shrimp is cooked through.
5. Serve hot over cooked quinoa.
6. Garnish with lemon slices.

Nutrition Information:

- Calories: 250
- Protein: 20g

- Carbohydrates: 25g

- Fat: 8g

- Fiber: 4g

- Sugar: 3g

- Portion size: 2 skewers with quinoa

Veggie Stir-Fry with Tofu

Ingredients:

- 1 block firm tofu, cubed

- 2 cups mixed vegetables (broccoli, bell peppers, snap peas, carrots)

- 2 tablespoons soy sauce

- 1 tablespoon hoisin sauce

- 1 tablespoon sesame oil

- 2 cloves garlic, minced

- 1 teaspoon ginger, grated

- Cooked brown rice for serving

Instructions:

1. Heat sesame oil in a large skillet over medium-high heat.

2. Add cubed tofu to the skillet, cook until golden brown on all sides.

3. Remove tofu from the skillet and set aside.

4. In the same skillet, add minced garlic and grated ginger, cook until fragrant.

5. Add mixed vegetables to the skillet, stir-fry for 3-4 minutes.

6. Return tofu to the skillet, drizzle soy sauce and hoisin sauce over the mixture.

7. Cook for another 2-3 minutes until heated through.

8. Serve hot over cooked brown rice.

Nutrition Information:

- Calories: 280
- Protein: 18g
- Carbohydrates: 30g
- Fat: 10g
- Fiber: 6g
- Sugar: 8g
- Portion size: 1 cup of stir-fry with tofu and rice

Chicken and Vegetable Kebabs

Ingredients:

- 1 lb boneless, skinless chicken breasts, cut into cubes
- 2 bell peppers, cut into chunks
- 1 red onion, cut into chunks
- 1 zucchini, sliced
- 1/4 cup olive oil
- 2 tablespoons lemon juice
- 2 cloves garlic, minced
- 1 teaspoon dried oregano
- Salt and pepper to taste
- Wooden skewers, soaked in water

Instructions:

1. In a bowl, whisk together olive oil, lemon juice, minced garlic, dried oregano, salt, and pepper to make the marinade.
2. Thread chicken cubes, bell pepper chunks, onion chunks, and zucchini slices onto the wooden skewers.
3. Place the skewers in a shallow dish and pour the marinade over them. Turn to coat evenly.

4. Cover and refrigerate for at least 30 minutes or up to
    2 hours.
5. Preheat the grill to medium-high heat.
6. Grill the kebabs for 8-10 minutes, turning
    occasionally, until chicken is cooked through and
    vegetables are tender.
7. Serve hot.

Nutrition Information:

- Calories: 280
- Protein: 25g
- Carbohydrates: 10g
- Fat: 15g
- Fiber: 3g
- Sugar: 5g
- Portion size: 2 kebabs

Black Bean and Corn Quesadillas

Ingredients:

- 4 whole wheat tortillas
- 1 can black beans, drained and rinsed
- 1 cup frozen corn kernels, thawed

- 1 cup shredded cheddar cheese
- 1/2 cup salsa
- 1 avocado, sliced
- Cooking spray

Instructions:

1. In a bowl, mix together black beans, corn kernels, shredded cheddar cheese, and salsa.
2. Heat a non-stick skillet over medium heat.
3. Place a tortilla in the skillet and spread a quarter of the bean and corn mixture over half of the tortilla.
4. Top with a few slices of avocado and fold the tortilla in half.
5. Cook for 2-3 minutes on each side until golden brown and cheese is melted.
6. Repeat with the remaining tortillas and filling.
7. Slice each quesadilla into wedges and serve hot.

Nutrition Information:

- Calories: 300
- Protein: 15g
- Carbohydrates: 30g

- Fat: 15g
- Fiber: 8g
- Sugar: 3g
- Portion size: 1 quesadilla

Turkey Meatballs with Zucchini Noodles

Ingredients:

- 1 lb ground turkey
- 1/2 cup breadcrumbs
- 1 egg
- 2 cloves garlic, minced
- 1 teaspoon Italian seasoning
- Salt and pepper to taste
- 2 zucchinis, spiralized into noodles
- 1 cup marinara sauce
- Fresh basil leaves for garnish

Instructions:

1. In a bowl, mix together ground turkey, breadcrumbs, egg, minced garlic, Italian seasoning, salt, and pepper.
2. Roll the mixture into meatballs of equal size.
3. Heat a non-stick skillet over medium heat and add the meatballs.
4. Cook for 8-10 minutes, turning occasionally, until browned and cooked through.
5. In the same skillet, add spiralized zucchini noodles and marinara sauce.
6. Cook for 3-4 minutes until noodles are heated through.
7. Serve turkey meatballs over zucchini noodles.
8. Garnish with fresh basil leaves.

Nutrition Information:

- Calories: 250
- Protein: 20g
- Carbohydrates: 15g
- Fat: 10g
- Fiber: 3g

- Sugar: 5g
- Portion size: 3 meatballs with zucchini noodles

Hawaiian Chicken Kabobs

Ingredients:

- 1 lb chicken breast, cut into chunks
- 1 cup pineapple chunks
- 1 bell pepper, cut into chunks
- 1 red onion, cut into chunks
- 1/4 cup soy sauce
- 2 tablespoons honey
- 2 tablespoons olive oil
- 1 teaspoon garlic powder
- Salt and pepper to taste
- Wooden skewers, soaked in water

Instructions:

1. In a bowl, whisk together soy sauce, honey, olive oil, garlic powder, salt, and pepper to make the marinade.

2. Thread chicken chunks, pineapple chunks, bell pepper chunks, and red onion chunks onto the wooden skewers.

3. Place the skewers in a shallow dish and pour the marinade over them. Turn to coat evenly.

4. Cover and refrigerate for at least 30 minutes or up to 2 hours.

5. Preheat the grill to medium-high heat.

6. Grill the kabobs for 8-10 minutes, turning occasionally, until chicken is cooked through and vegetables are tender.

7. Serve hot over cooked rice or quinoa.

Nutrition Information:

- Calories: 280
- Protein: 25g
- Carbohydrates: 20g
- Fat: 10g
- Fiber: 3g
- Sugar: 15g
- Portion size: 2 kabobs

Lentil and Sweet Potato Curry

Ingredients:

- 1 cup dried lentils, rinsed

- 2 sweet potatoes, peeled and diced
- 1 onion, diced
- 2 cloves garlic, minced
- 1 can coconut milk
- 1 can diced tomatoes
- 2 tablespoons curry powder
- 1 teaspoon turmeric
- Salt and pepper to taste
- Fresh cilantro for garnish

Instructions:

1. In a large pot, combine lentils, diced sweet potatoes, diced onion, minced garlic, coconut milk, diced tomatoes, curry powder, turmeric, salt, and pepper.
2. Bring to a boil over medium-high heat.
3. Reduce heat to low, cover, and simmer for 20-25 minutes until lentils and sweet potatoes are tender.
4. Serve hot, garnished with fresh cilantro.
5. Optional: Serve over cooked brown rice or quinoa.

Nutrition Information:

- Calories: 300

- Protein: 15g

- Carbohydrates: 40g

- Fat: 10g

- Fiber: 12g

- Sugar: 10g

- Portion size: 1 cup

Baked Cod with Tomato and Basil

Ingredients:

- 4 cod fillets

- 2 cups cherry tomatoes, halved

- 1/4 cup fresh basil leaves, chopped

- 2 cloves garlic, minced

- 2 tablespoons olive oil

- Salt and pepper to taste

- Lemon wedges for serving

Instructions:

1. Preheat the oven to 400°F (200°C).

2. Place cod fillets in a baking dish.

3. In a bowl, toss together cherry tomatoes, chopped basil, minced garlic, olive oil, salt, and pepper.

4. Spoon the tomato mixture over the cod fillets.

5. Bake for 15-20 minutes until cod is cooked through and tomatoes are softened.

6. Serve hot with lemon wedges.

Nutrition Information:

- Calories: 250

- Protein: 25g

- Carbohydrates: 10g

- Fat: 10g

- Fiber: 3g

- Sugar: 5g

- Portion size: 1 cod fillet with tomato mixture

Chapter 5: Snacks and Appetizers

In this chapter, we've curated a selection of wholesome snacks and appetizers that are perfect for kids with diabetes. Each recipe is packed with flavor and carefully balanced to provide essential nutrients without causing spikes in blood sugar.

Hummus with Carrot and Celery Sticks

Ingredients:

- 1 cup chickpeas (canned, drained, and rinsed)
- 2 tablespoons tahini
- 2 tablespoons lemon juice
- 1 clove garlic, minced
- 2 tablespoons olive oil
- Salt and pepper to taste
- Carrot and celery sticks for dipping

Instructions:

1. In a food processor, combine chickpeas, tahini, lemon juice, garlic, olive oil, salt, and pepper.
2. Blend until smooth and creamy, scraping down the sides as needed.
3. Transfer the hummus to a serving bowl and refrigerate for at least 30 minutes before serving.
4. Serve with carrot and celery sticks for dipping.

Nutrition Information (per serving):

- Calories: 120
- Protein: 4g
- Carbohydrates: 10g
- Fat: 7g
- Fiber: 3g
- Sugar: 2g
- Portion size: 2 tablespoons hummus with 1 cup carrot and celery sticks

Greek Yogurt Dip with Fresh Veggies

Ingredients:

- 1 cup Greek yogurt
- 1 tablespoon lemon juice
- 1 teaspoon dried dill
- 1/2 teaspoon garlic powder
- Salt and pepper to taste
- Assorted fresh veggies for dipping (such as cucumber slices, cherry tomatoes, bell pepper strips)

Instructions:

1. In a small bowl, mix together Greek yogurt, lemon juice, dried dill, garlic powder, salt, and pepper.
2. Stir until well combined.
3. Refrigerate for at least 30 minutes to allow the flavors to meld.
4. Serve with fresh veggies for dipping.

Nutrition Information (per serving):

- Calories: 60
- Protein: 6g

- Carbohydrates: 5g
- Fat: 2g
- Fiber: 1g
- Sugar: 3g
- Portion size: 1/4 cup dip with assorted veggies

Cheese and Whole Grain Crackers

Ingredients:

- Whole grain crackers
- Slices of your favorite cheese (such as cheddar, mozzarella, or Swiss)

Instructions:

1. Arrange whole grain crackers on a serving platter.
2. Top each cracker with a slice of cheese.
3. Serve immediately.

Nutrition Information (per serving):

- Calories: 80
- Protein: 5g
- Carbohydrates: 10g
- Fat: 3g

- Fiber: 2g

- Sugar: 1g

- Portion size: 5 whole grain crackers with 1 slice of cheese

Apple Slices with Almond Butter

Ingredients:

- 1 apple, sliced

- 2 tablespoons almond butter

Instructions:

1. Arrange apple slices on a plate.

2. Serve with almond butter for dipping.

Nutrition Information (per serving):

- Calories: 150

- Protein: 4g

- Carbohydrates: 20g

- Fat: 8g

- Fiber: 5g

- Sugar: 14g

- Portion size: 1 medium apple with 2 tablespoons almond butter

Trail Mix with Nuts and Dried Fruit

Ingredients:

- 1/4 cup almonds
- 1/4 cup cashews
- 1/4 cup dried cranberries
- 1/4 cup raisins
- 1/4 cup dark chocolate chips

Instructions:

1. In a bowl, combine almonds, cashews, dried cranberries, raisins, and dark chocolate chips.
2. Toss until evenly mixed.
3. Divide into individual portions and store in an airtight container for easy snacking.

Nutrition Information (per serving):

- Calories: 200
- Protein: 5g
- Carbohydrates: 25g

- Fat: 10g

- Fiber: 3g

- Sugar: 15g

- Portion size: 1/4 cup trail mix

Cottage Cheese with Pineapple Chunks

Ingredients:

- 1/2 cup low-fat cottage cheese

- 1/2 cup pineapple chunks (fresh or canned in juice)

Instructions:

1. Spoon cottage cheese into a serving bowl.
2. Top with pineapple chunks.
3. Serve chilled.

Nutrition Information (per serving):

- Calories: 120

- Protein: 14g

- Carbohydrates: 15g

- Fat: 2g

- Fiber: 1g
- Sugar: 10g
- Portion size: 1/2 cup cottage cheese with 1/2 cup pineapple chunks

Edamame with Sea Salt

Ingredients:

- 1 cup edamame (frozen, thawed)
- Sea salt to taste

Instructions:

1. Steam or boil edamame according to package instructions.
2. Drain and sprinkle with sea salt.
3. Serve warm or chilled.

Nutrition Information (per serving):

- Calories: 100
- Protein: 9g
- Carbohydrates: 8g
- Fat: 4g
- Fiber: 4g

- Sugar: 1g
- Portion size: 1 cup edamame

Guacamole and Baked Tortilla Chips

Ingredients:

- 2 ripe avocados
- 1 small tomato, diced
- 1/4 cup red onion, finely chopped
- 1 tablespoon lime juice
- 1 clove garlic, minced
- Salt and pepper to taste
- Baked tortilla chips for serving

Instructions:

1. In a bowl, mash the avocados with a fork until smooth.
2. Stir in diced tomato, chopped red onion, lime juice, minced garlic, salt, and pepper.
3. Mix until well combined.
4. Serve with baked tortilla chips for dipping.

Nutrition Information (per serving):

- Calories: 150
- Protein: 2g
- Carbohydrates: 10g
- Fat: 12g
- Fiber: 6g
- Sugar: 1g
- Portion size: 1/4 cup guacamole with 10 baked tortilla chips

Cucumber and Tomato Salad

Ingredients:

- 1 cucumber, diced
- 1 cup cherry tomatoes, halved
- 2 tablespoons red onion, finely chopped
- 1 tablespoon fresh parsley, chopped
- 1 tablespoon olive oil
- 1 tablespoon red wine vinegar
- Salt and pepper to taste

Instructions:

1. In a bowl, combine diced cucumber, halved cherry tomatoes, chopped red onion, and chopped parsley.
2. Drizzle with olive oil and red wine vinegar.
3. Season with salt and pepper.
4. Toss until evenly coated.
5. Serve chilled.

Nutrition Information (per serving):

- Calories: 60
- Protein: 1g
- Carbohydrates: 5g
- Fat: 4g
- Fiber: 1g
- Sugar: 2g
- Portion size: 1 cup salad

Ants on a Log (Celery with Peanut Butter and Raisins)

Ingredients:

- Celery stalks, cut into sticks

- Peanut butter
- Raisins

Instructions:

1. Spread peanut butter onto celery sticks.
2. Press raisins onto the peanut butter.
3. Serve immediately.

Nutrition Information (per serving):

- Calories: 100
- Protein: 3g
- Carbohydrates: 8g
- Fat: 6g
- Fiber: 2g
- Sugar: 4g
- Portion size: 2 celery sticks with peanut butter and raisins

Roasted Chickpeas with Seasonings

Ingredients:

- 1 can (15 ounces) chickpeas, drained and rinsed
- 1 tablespoon olive oil

- 1 teaspoon ground cumin
- 1/2 teaspoon smoked paprika
- 1/2 teaspoon garlic powder
- Salt to taste

Instructions:

1. Preheat the oven to 400°F (200°C).
2. Pat the chickpeas dry with a paper towel and spread them on a baking sheet.
3. Drizzle with olive oil and sprinkle with cumin, smoked paprika, garlic powder, and salt.
4. Toss until the chickpeas are evenly coated.
5. Roast in the preheated oven for 20-25 minutes, stirring halfway through, until crispy.
6. Let cool before serving.

Nutrition Information (per serving):

- Calories: 150
- Protein: 6g
- Carbohydrates: 20g
- Fat: 5g
- Fiber: 6g

- Sugar: 4g
- Portion size: 1/2 cup roasted chickpeas

Avocado Deviled Eggs

Ingredients:

- 6 hard-boiled eggs, peeled and halved
- 1 ripe avocado
- 1 tablespoon lime juice
- 1/2 teaspoon Dijon mustard
- Salt and pepper to taste
- Paprika for garnish

Instructions:

1. Remove the yolks from the halved eggs and place them in a bowl.
2. Mash the yolks with avocado, lime juice, Dijon mustard, salt, and pepper until smooth.
3. Spoon the avocado mixture into the egg white halves.
4. Sprinkle with paprika for garnish.
5. Serve chilled.

Nutrition Information (per serving):

- Calories: 100
- Protein: 6g
- Carbohydrates: 3g
- Fat: 7g
- Fiber: 2g
- Sugar: 0g
- Portion size: 2 avocado deviled egg halves

Whole Grain Pita Chips with Salsa

Ingredients:

- Whole grain pita bread
- Olive oil spray
- Salt to taste
- Salsa for dipping

Instructions:

1. Preheat the oven to 350°F (175°C).
2. Cut the pita bread into wedges and place them on a baking sheet.
3. Lightly spray the pita wedges with olive oil and sprinkle with salt.

4. Bake in the preheated oven for 8-10 minutes, or until crispy and golden brown.

5. Let cool before serving with salsa for dipping.

Nutrition Information (per serving):

- Calories: 120

- Protein: 3g

- Carbohydrates: 20g

- Fat: 3g

- Fiber: 4g

- Sugar: 2g

- Portion size: 6 pita chips with salsa

Turkey and Cheese Kabobs

Ingredients:

- 4 slices turkey breast, cut into cubes

- 4 slices cheese (such as cheddar or Swiss), cut into cubes

- Cherry tomatoes

- Cucumber, cut into chunks

- Wooden skewers

Instructions:

1. Thread turkey cubes, cheese cubes, cherry tomatoes, and cucumber chunks onto wooden skewers in alternating patterns.
2. Repeat until all ingredients are used.
3. Serve immediately or refrigerate until ready to serve.

Nutrition Information (per serving):

- Calories: 150
- Protein: 12g
- Carbohydrates: 3g
- Fat: 10g
- Fiber: 1g
- Sugar: 1g
- Portion size: 2 kabobs

Almond Butter Energy Bites

Ingredients:

- 1 cup rolled oats
- 1/2 cup almond butter
- 1/4 cup honey or maple syrup
- 1/4 cup dark chocolate chips

- 1/4 cup shredded coconut (optional)
- 1 teaspoon vanilla extract

Instructions:

1. In a mixing bowl, combine rolled oats, almond butter, honey or maple syrup, dark chocolate chips, shredded coconut (if using), and vanilla extract.
2. Mix until well combined.
3. Roll the mixture into small balls using your hands.
4. Place the energy bites on a baking sheet lined with parchment paper.
5. Refrigerate for at least 30 minutes before serving.

Nutrition Information (per serving):

- Calories: 120
- Protein: 4g
- Carbohydrates: 15g
- Fat: 6g
- Fiber: 2g
- Sugar: 7g
- Portion size: 2 energy bites

Chapter 6: Desserts

In this chapter, you'll find a collection of Desserts designed to please young palates while providing essential nutrients to keep them energized and satisfied. From fruity delights to creamy indulgences, these recipes offer a balance of flavors and textures that make snack time a joyous occasion.

Banana Ice Cream with Dark Chocolate Chips

Ingredients:

- 2 ripe bananas
- 1/4 cup dark chocolate chips

Instructions:

1. Peel the bananas and slice them into coins.
2. Place the banana slices in a single layer on a baking sheet lined with parchment paper.
3. Freeze the banana slices for at least 2 hours or until frozen solid.

4. Once frozen, transfer the banana slices to a blender or food processor.

5. Blend the banana slices until smooth and creamy, scraping down the sides as needed.

6. Add the dark chocolate chips to the blender and pulse a few times to combine.

7. Serve immediately as soft-serve ice cream or transfer to a container and freeze for a firmer texture.

Nutrition Information (per serving):

- Calories: 150
- Protein: 2g
- Carbohydrates: 25g
- Fat: 6g
- Fiber: 3g
- Sugar: 14g
- Portion Size: 1/2 cup

Baked Apple Chips

Ingredients:

- 2 apples
- Cinnamon (optional)

Instructions:

1. Preheat the oven to 200°F (95°C) and line a baking sheet with parchment paper.
2. Wash and core the apples, then slice them thinly using a sharp knife or mandoline.
3. Arrange the apple slices in a single layer on the prepared baking sheet.
4. Sprinkle with cinnamon if desired.
5. Bake for 1.5 to 2 hours, flipping the apple slices halfway through, until they are dried and crisp.
6. Allow the apple chips to cool completely before serving.

Nutrition Information (per serving):

- Calories: 50
- Protein: 0g
- Carbohydrates: 13g
- Fat: 0g
- Fiber: 3g
- Sugar: 10g
- Portion Size: 1/2 apple

Berry Yogurt Popsicles

Ingredients:

- 1 cup mixed berries (strawberries, blueberries, raspberries)
- 1 cup plain yogurt
- 2 tablespoons honey (optional)

Instructions:

1. In a blender, combine the mixed berries, yogurt, and honey (if using).
2. Blend until smooth.
3. Pour the mixture into popsicle molds.
4. Insert popsicle sticks and freeze for at least 4 hours or until firm.
5. Run the molds under warm water for a few seconds to release the popsicles.
6. Serve immediately or store in the freezer for later enjoyment.

Nutrition Information (per serving):

- Calories: 60
- Protein: 3g

- Carbohydrates: 12g

- Fat: 1g

- Fiber: 2g

- Sugar: 9g

- Portion Size: 1 popsicle

Chocolate Avocado Mousse

Ingredients:

- 2 ripe avocados

- 1/4 cup cocoa powder

- 1/4 cup honey or maple syrup

- 1 teaspoon vanilla extract

Instructions:

1. Scoop the flesh of the avocados into a blender or food processor.

2. Add cocoa powder, honey or maple syrup, and vanilla extract.

3. Blend until smooth and creamy, scraping down the sides as needed.

4. Divide the mousse into serving cups and chill in the refrigerator for at least 30 minutes before serving.

Nutrition Information (per serving):

- Calories: 150
- Protein: 2g
- Carbohydrates: 17g
- Fat: 10g
- Fiber: 6g
- Sugar: 9g
- Portion Size: 1/2 cup

Frozen Grapes

Ingredients:

- Seedless grapes

Instructions:

1. Rinse the grapes and remove them from the stems.
2. Pat the grapes dry with a paper towel.
3. Place the grapes in a single layer on a baking sheet lined with parchment paper.
4. Freeze for at least 2 hours or until firm.
5. Serve the frozen grapes as a refreshing and naturally sweet snack.

Nutrition Information (per serving):

- Calories: 60
- Protein: 1g
- Carbohydrates: 15g
- Fat: 0g
- Fiber: 1g
- Sugar: 12g
- Portion Size: 1 cup

Mini Fruit Tartlets

Ingredients:

- Mini tart shells
- Assorted fresh fruits (such as berries, kiwi, and mango)
- 1/2 cup Greek yogurt
- 1 tablespoon honey
- Fresh mint leaves for garnish (optional)

Instructions:

1. In a small bowl, mix Greek yogurt with honey until well combined.
2. Spoon the yogurt mixture into the mini tart shells.

3. Top each tartlet with assorted fresh fruits.

4. Garnish with fresh mint leaves if desired.

5. Chill in the refrigerator until ready to serve.

Nutrition Information (per serving):

- Calories: 80

- Protein: 2g

- Carbohydrates: 15g

- Fat: 2g

- Fiber: 1g

- Sugar: 10g

- Portion Size: 1 tartlet

Pumpkin Spice Energy Balls

Ingredients:

- 1 cup rolled oats

- 1/2 cup pumpkin puree

- 1/4 cup almond butter

- 2 tablespoons maple syrup

- 1 teaspoon pumpkin pie spice

- 1/4 cup shredded coconut (optional)

Instructions:

1. In a mixing bowl, combine rolled oats, pumpkin puree, almond butter, maple syrup, and pumpkin pie spice.
2. Mix until well combined.
3. Roll the mixture into small balls using your hands.
4. Optional: Roll the balls in shredded coconut for added texture.
5. Refrigerate for at least 30 minutes before serving.

Nutrition Information (per serving):

- Calories: 80
- Protein: 2g
- Carbohydrates: 10g
- Fat: 4g
- Fiber: 2g
- Sugar: 3g
- Portion Size: 1 energy ball

Strawberry Banana Smoothie Bowl

Ingredients:

- 1 cup frozen strawberries

- 1 ripe banana
- 1/2 cup plain Greek yogurt
- 1/4 cup almond milk (or any milk of choice)
- Toppings: sliced banana, fresh strawberries, granola, chia seeds

Instructions:

1. In a blender, combine frozen strawberries, banana, Greek yogurt, and almond milk.
2. Blend until smooth and creamy.
3. Pour the smoothie into a bowl.
4. Top with sliced banana, fresh strawberries, granola, and chia seeds.
5. Serve immediately.

Nutrition Information (per serving):

- Calories: 150
- Protein: 7g
- Carbohydrates: 30g
- Fat: 2g
- Fiber: 6g
- Sugar: 18g

- Portion Size: 1 bowl

Yogurt-Dipped Strawberries

Ingredients:

- Fresh strawberries
- Greek yogurt
- Honey (optional)
- Sprinkles (optional)

Instructions:

1. Wash and dry the strawberries, leaving the stems intact.
2. In a small bowl, mix Greek yogurt with honey if desired.
3. Dip each strawberry into the yogurt mixture, coating about halfway.
4. Optional: Roll the yogurt-covered portion of the strawberries in sprinkles for added fun.
5. Place the strawberries on a baking sheet lined with parchment paper.
6. Freeze for about 30 minutes or until the yogurt is set.
7. Serve chilled.

Nutrition Information (per serving):

- Calories: 40
- Protein: 2g
- Carbohydrates: 7g
- Fat: 0g
- Fiber: 1g
- Sugar: 5g
- Portion Size: 3 strawberries

Peach Frozen Yogurt

Ingredients:

- 2 cups frozen peach slices
- 1/2 cup plain Greek yogurt
- 2 tablespoons honey or maple syrup

Instructions:

1. In a blender or food processor, combine the frozen peach slices, Greek yogurt, and honey or maple syrup.
2. Blend until smooth and creamy, scraping down the sides as needed.
3. Transfer the mixture to a freezer-safe container.

4. Freeze for at least 2 hours or until firm.

5. Allow the frozen yogurt to soften slightly at room temperature before serving.

Nutrition Information (per serving):

- Calories: 100

- Protein: 4g

- Carbohydrates: 22g

- Fat: 0g

- Fiber: 3g

- Sugar: 18g

- Portion Size: 1/2 cup

Blueberry Chia Seed Popsicles

Ingredients:

- 1 cup blueberries

- 1 cup unsweetened almond milk

- 2 tablespoons chia seeds

- 1 tablespoon honey or maple syrup (optional)

Instructions:

1. In a blender, combine the blueberries, almond milk, chia seeds, and honey or maple syrup (if using).

2. Blend until smooth.

3. Pour the mixture into popsicle molds.

4. Insert popsicle sticks and freeze for at least 4 hours or until firm.

5. Run the molds under warm water for a few seconds to release the popsicles.

6. Serve immediately.

Nutrition Information (per serving):

- Calories: 50
- Protein: 1g
- Carbohydrates: 9g
- Fat: 2g
- Fiber: 3g
- Sugar: 5g
- Portion Size: 1 popsicle

Watermelon Pizza with Yogurt and Fruit Toppings

Ingredients:

- 1/2 small watermelon, sliced into rounds
- Plain Greek yogurt
- Assorted fruits (such as berries, kiwi, and grapes)
- Fresh mint leaves for garnish (optional)

Instructions:

1. Place the watermelon rounds on a serving platter.
2. Spread a layer of Greek yogurt over each watermelon round.
3. Arrange assorted fruits on top of the yogurt.
4. Garnish with fresh mint leaves if desired.
5. Slice the watermelon pizza into wedges and serve immediately.

Nutrition Information (per serving):

- Calories: 60
- Protein: 2g
- Carbohydrates: 13g
- Fat: 0g

- Fiber: 1g
- Sugar: 10g
- Portion Size: 1 slice

Mango Sorbet

Ingredients:

- 2 cups frozen mango chunks
- 1/4 cup coconut water
- 1 tablespoon lime juice
- 2 tablespoons honey or maple syrup (optional)

Instructions:

1. In a blender or food processor, combine the frozen mango chunks, coconut water, lime juice, and honey or maple syrup (if using).
2. Blend until smooth and creamy, scraping down the sides as needed.
3. Transfer the mixture to a freezer-safe container.
4. Freeze for at least 2 hours or until firm.
5. Allow the sorbet to soften slightly at room temperature before serving.

Nutrition Information (per serving):

- Calories: 90
- Protein: 1g
- Carbohydrates: 24g
- Fat: 0g
- Fiber: 2g
- Sugar: 22g
- Portion Size: 1/2 cup

Kiwi and Berry Parfait

Ingredients:

- 2 kiwis, peeled and diced
- 1 cup mixed berries (such as strawberries, blueberries, raspberries)
- 1 cup plain Greek yogurt
- 1/4 cup granola

Instructions:

1. In serving glasses or bowls, layer diced kiwis, mixed berries, and Greek yogurt.
2. Repeat the layers until the glasses are filled.
3. Top each parfait with granola.

4. Serve immediately.

Nutrition Information (per serving):

- Calories: 120
- Protein: 7g
- Carbohydrates: 20g
- Fat: 2g
- Fiber: 4g
- Sugar: 12g
- Portion Size: 1 parfait

Coconut Almond Date Bites

Ingredients:

- 1 cup pitted dates
- 1/2 cup almonds
- 1/4 cup unsweetened shredded coconut
- 1 tablespoon coconut oil
- 1/2 teaspoon vanilla extract

Instructions:

1. In a food processor, combine dates, almonds, shredded coconut, coconut oil, and vanilla extract.

2. Pulse until the mixture comes together and forms a sticky dough.

3. Roll the dough into small balls using your hands.

4. Optional: Roll the balls in additional shredded coconut for coating.

5. Refrigerate for at least 30 minutes before serving.

Nutrition Information (per serving):

- Calories: 80

- Protein: 2g

- Carbohydrates: 10g

- Fat: 4g

- Fiber: 2g

- Sugar: 8g

- Portion Size: 2 bites

Chapter 7: Smoothies

These delightful concoctions are not only delicious but also packed with essential nutrients to keep you energized throughout the day. From vibrant greens to luscious fruits, each smoothie recipe offers a unique blend of flavors and health benefits. So, grab your blender and let's blend up some goodness!

Green Power Smoothie with Spinach and Kale

Ingredients:

- 1 cup spinach
- 1 cup kale
- 1 banana
- 1/2 cup pineapple chunks
- 1/2 cup almond milk

Instructions:

1. Add all ingredients to a blender.
2. Blend until smooth.

3. Pour into a glass and enjoy!

Nutrition Information:

- Calories: 150

- Protein: 5g

- Carbohydrates: 30g

- Fat: 2g

- Fiber: 7g

- Sugar: 15g

- Portion size: 1 serving

Berry Blast Smoothie

Ingredients:

- 1 cup mixed berries (strawberries, blueberries, raspberries)

- 1/2 cup Greek yogurt

- 1/2 cup almond milk

- 1 tablespoon honey (optional)

Instructions:

1. Combine all ingredients in a blender.

2. Blend until smooth.

3. Serve and enjoy!

Nutrition Information:

- Calories: 180

- Protein: 10g

- Carbohydrates: 30g

- Fat: 3g

- Fiber: 6g

- Sugar: 20g

- Portion size: 1 serving

Banana Peanut Butter Smoothie

Ingredients:

- 1 ripe banana

- 2 tablespoons peanut butter

- 1 cup almond milk

- 1 tablespoon honey (optional)

Instructions:

1. Place all ingredients in a blender.

2. Blend until creamy and smooth.

3. Pour into a glass and enjoy!

Nutrition Information:

- Calories: 280
- Protein: 8g
- Carbohydrates: 30g
- Fat: 15g
- Fiber: 5g
- Sugar: 18g
- Portion size: 1 serving

Mango Tango Smoothie

Ingredients:

- 1 cup diced mango
- 1/2 cup plain Greek yogurt
- 1/2 cup orange juice
- 1/2 cup ice cubes

Instructions:

1. Add all ingredients to a blender.
2. Blend until smooth and creamy.
3. Pour into a glass and enjoy!

Nutrition Information:

- Calories: 200
- Protein: 10g
- Carbohydrates: 40g
- Fat: 1g
- Fiber: 3g
- Sugar: 35g
- Portion size: 1 serving

Pineapple Paradise Smoothie

Ingredients:

- 1 cup diced pineapple
- 1/2 cup coconut milk
- 1/2 cup spinach
- 1 tablespoon chia seeds

Instructions:

1. Place all ingredients in a blender.
2. Blend until smooth and creamy.
3. Pour into a glass and enjoy!

Nutrition Information:

- Calories: 220
- Protein: 5g
- Carbohydrates: 30g
- Fat: 10g
- Fiber: 8g
- Sugar: 15g
- Portion size: 1 serving

Chocolate Banana Protein Smoothie

Ingredients:

- 1 ripe banana
- 1 scoop chocolate protein powder
- 1 cup almond milk
- 1 tablespoon cocoa powder

Instructions:

1. Combine all ingredients in a blender.
2. Blend until smooth and creamy.
3. Pour into a glass and enjoy!

Nutrition Information:

- Calories: 250
- Protein: 20g
- Carbohydrates: 30g
- Fat: 5g
- Fiber: 6g
- Sugar: 15g
- Portion size: 1 serving

Tropical Sunrise Smoothie

Ingredients:

- 1/2 cup diced pineapple
- 1/2 cup diced mango
- 1/2 cup orange juice
- 1/2 cup coconut water

Instructions:

1. Add all ingredients to a blender.
2. Blend until smooth and creamy.
3. Serve immediately and enjoy!

Nutrition Information:

- Calories: 180
- Protein: 2g
- Carbohydrates: 40g
- Fat: 1g
- Fiber: 4g
- Sugar: 30g
- Portion size: 1 serving

Kiwi Kale Smoothie

Ingredients:

- 2 kiwis, peeled and sliced
- 1 cup kale leaves
- 1/2 cup green grapes
- 1/2 cup coconut water

Instructions:

1. Place all ingredients in a blender.
2. Blend until smooth and creamy.
3. Pour into glasses and serve immediately.

Nutrition Information:

- Calories: 160
- Protein: 4g
- Carbohydrates: 35g
- Fat: 1g
- Fiber: 7g
- Sugar: 20g
- Portion size: 1 serving

Peach Raspberry Smoothie

Ingredients:

- 1 cup sliced peaches
- 1/2 cup raspberries
- 1/2 cup plain Greek yogurt
- 1/2 cup almond milk

Instructions:

1. Add all ingredients to a blender.
2. Blend until smooth and creamy.
3. Pour into glasses and serve immediately.

Nutrition Information:

- Calories: 170
- Protein: 8g
- Carbohydrates: 30g
- Fat: 3g
- Fiber: 6g
- Sugar: 20g
- Portion size: 1 serving

Avocado Spinach Smoothie

Ingredients:

- 1/2 ripe avocado
- 1 cup spinach
- 1/2 cup sliced cucumber
- 1/2 cup coconut water

Instructions:

1. Combine all ingredients in a blender.
2. Blend until smooth and creamy.
3. Pour into glasses and serve immediately.

Nutrition Information:

- Calories: 200
- Protein: 5g
- Carbohydrates: 25g
- Fat: 10g
- Fiber: 8g
- Sugar: 10g
- Portion size: 1 serving

Blueberry Almond Smoothie

Ingredients:

- 1 cup blueberries
- 1/4 cup almonds
- 1/2 cup Greek yogurt
- 1/2 cup almond milk

Instructions:

1. Add all ingredients to a blender.
2. Blend until smooth and creamy.
3. Pour into glasses and enjoy!

Nutrition Information:

- Calories: 220
- Protein: 10g
- Carbohydrates: 30g
- Fat: 8g
- Fiber: 6g
- Sugar: 15g
- Portion size: 1 serving

Orange Creamsicle Smoothie

Ingredients:

- 1 cup orange juice
- 1/2 cup Greek yogurt
- 1/2 cup ice cubes
- 1 tablespoon honey (optional)

Instructions:

1. Combine all ingredients in a blender.
2. Blend until smooth and creamy.
3. Serve immediately and enjoy!

Nutrition Information:

- Calories: 160
- Protein: 8g
- Carbohydrates: 35g
- Fat: 1g
- Fiber: 3g
- Sugar: 25g
- Portion size: 1 serving

Mixed Berry Oatmeal Smoothie

Ingredients:

- 1/2 cup mixed berries
- 1/4 cup rolled oats
- 1/2 cup Greek yogurt
- 1/2 cup almond milk

Instructions:

1. Add all ingredients to a blender.
2. Blend until smooth and creamy.
3. Pour into glasses and enjoy!

Nutrition Information:

- Calories: 210
- Protein: 10g
- Carbohydrates: 35g
- Fat: 4g
- Fiber: 7g
- Sugar: 15g
- Portion size: 1 serving

Peanut Butter and Jelly Smoothie

Ingredients:

- 2 tablespoons peanut butter
- 1/2 cup strawberries
- 1/2 cup grapes
- 1/2 cup almond milk

Instructions:

1. Combine all ingredients in a blender.
2. Blend until smooth and creamy.
3. Pour into glasses and serve immediately.

Nutrition Information:

- Calories: 240
- Protein: 8g
- Carbohydrates: 30g
- Fat: 12g
- Fiber: 5g
- Sugar: 18g
- Portion size: 1 serving

Cucumber Mint Smoothie

Ingredients:

- 1 cucumber, peeled and sliced
- 1/4 cup fresh mint leaves
- 1/2 cup Greek yogurt
- 1/2 cup coconut water

Instructions:

1. Add all ingredients to a blender.
2. Blend until smooth and creamy.
3. Pour into glasses and serve immediately.

Nutrition Information:

- Calories: 120
- Protein: 6g
- Carbohydrates: 20g
- Fat: 2g
- Fiber: 4g
- Sugar: 10g
- Portion size: 1 serving

CONCLUSION

As we reach the end of this journey through diabetes-friendly recipes tailored for children, it's essential to reflect on the significance of the culinary exploration we've undertaken together. Throughout this book, we've embarked on a flavorful adventure, blending nutritional expertise with creative cooking techniques to craft meals that nourish both body and soul.

Our goal was not just to provide a collection of recipes but to empower families with the knowledge and tools needed to manage diabetes effectively while enjoying a diverse and delicious diet. By embracing whole foods, balanced nutrition, and mindful eating habits, we've cultivated a culinary landscape where health and taste intertwine seamlessly.

Each recipe within these pages serves as a testament to the boundless possibilities of diabetic-friendly cooking. From vibrant breakfast bowls to hearty dinner entrees and tantalizing desserts, we've proven that managing blood sugar levels can be a joyous and fulfilling experience for both children and their families.

But beyond the kitchen, this book represents a journey of resilience, adaptation, and empowerment. It's a testament to the strength of families facing the challenges of diabetes head-on, transforming dietary restrictions into opportunities for creativity and growth. It's a celebration of the unwavering spirit of caregivers, who tirelessly strive to provide the best possible care for their loved ones.

As we bid farewell to these pages, let us carry forward the lessons learned and the flavors savored. Let us continue to explore, experiment, and innovate in the kitchen, armed with the knowledge that good nutrition is the cornerstone of well-being. And most importantly, let us remember that the true measure of success lies not in perfection but in progress, one wholesome meal at a time.

May this book serve as a beacon of hope, inspiration, and delicious possibility for all those navigating the complex landscape of childhood diabetes. Together, we've embarked on a journey towards better health, one recipe, one bite, and one smile at a time.

Bon appétit, and may your culinary adventures be as enriching as they are delectable.

www.ingramcontent.com/pod-product-compliance
Lightning Source LLC
Chambersburg PA
CBHW071012250726
48653CB00005B/1592